Simple Keto Recipe Book

Super Tasty and Delicious Dessert Recipes for Beginners

River Hunt

Blueberry Muffins

Cook Time:

30 minutes

Servings:6

Ingredients:

1 ½ cups flour

½ tsp salt

½ cup sugar

¼ cup vegetable oil

2 tsp vanilla extract

1 cup fresh blueberries

1 egg

2 tsp baking powder

Directions:

1.Preheat air fryer to 340 F. In a bowl, combine flour, salt, and baking powder.

2.In another bowl, add vegetable oil, vanilla extract, and egg and whisk the mixture until fully incorporated.

3.Combine the wet and dry ingredients; gently fold in the blueberries. Divide the mixture between a greased 6-hole muffin tray.

4.Bake in the air fryer for 10-12 minutes until set and golden. Serve cooled. Enjoy!

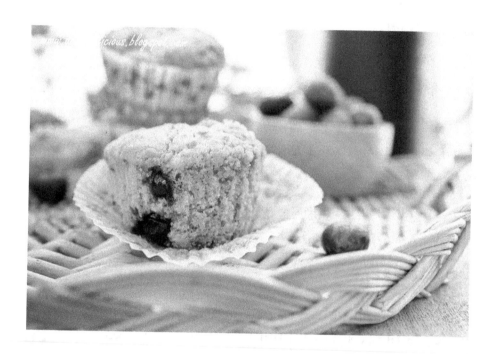

Orange Sponge Cake

Cook Time:

30 minutes

Servings:4

Ingredients:

1 cup sugar

1 cup self-rising flour

3 eggs

1 tsp vanilla extract

Zest and juice from 1 orange

2 egg whites

4 tbsp superfine sugar

½ cup ground walnuts

Directions:

1.Preheat air fryer to 360 F. In a bowl, beat sugar, flour, eggs, vanilla, and half of the orange zest with an electric mixer until creamy and fluffy, about 8 minutes.

2.Transfer half of the batter into a greased and floured cake pan and Bake in the air fryer for 15 minutes. Repeat the process for the remaining batter.

3.Meanwhile, prepare the frosting by beating egg whites, orange juice, and superfine sugar together.

4.Spread half of the frosting mixture on top of one cooled cake. Top with the other cake and spread the remaining frosting all over. Top with walnuts, slice, and serve. Enjoy!

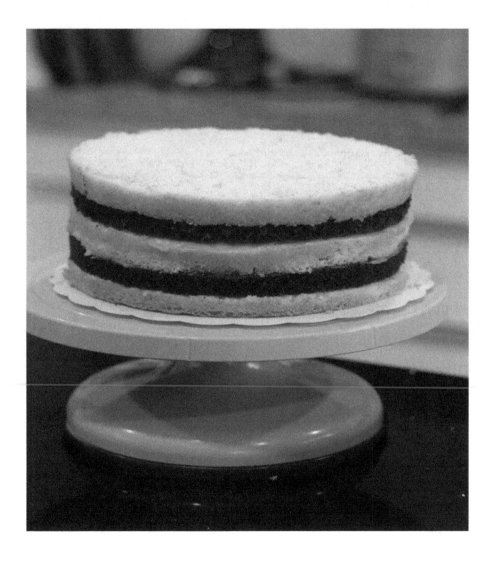

Lemon-Glazed Cupcakes

Cook Time:

30 minutes

Servings:6

Ingredients:

1 cup flour

½ cup sugar

1 egg

1 tsp lemon zest

¾ tsp baking powder

2 tbsp vegetable oil

½ cup milk

½ tsp vanilla extract

½ cup powdered sugar

2 tsp lemon juice

Directions:

1.Preheat air fryer to 360 F. In a bowl, combine flour, sugar, lemon zest, and baking powder.

2.In another bowl, whisk together egg, vegetable oil, milk, and vanilla extract. Gently combine the two mixtures to obtain a smooth batter.

3.Divide the batter between greased muffin tins or 6-hole muffin tray. Place the muffin tins or tray in the fryer and Bake for 12-14 minutes.

4.Remove muffins and let cool. 4.Whisk powdered sugar with lemon juice until smooth. Pour the glaze on top of the muffins and serve. Enjoy!

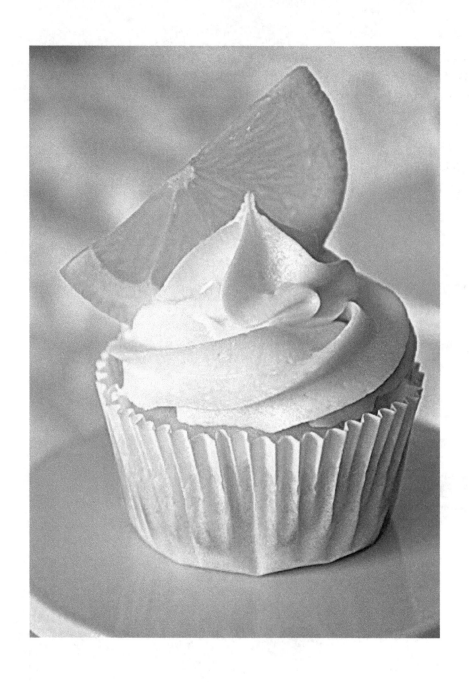

Air Fried Donuts

Cook Time:

30 minutes

Servings:4

Ingredients:

1 cup self-rising flour

1 tsp baking powder

½ cup milk

2 ½ tbsp butter, softened

1 egg, beaten

4 tbsp brown sugar

Directions:

1.Preheat air fryer to 350 F. In a bowl, whisk butter with brown sugar until smooth. Mix in eggs and milk to combine.

2.In another bowl, combine flour with baking powder. Fold the flour into the butter mixture.

3.Form donut shapes and cut off the center with cookie cutters. Arrange on a lined baking sheet and Bake in the fryer for 15 minutes.

4.Serve with whipped cream or drizzled with maple syrup. Enjoy!

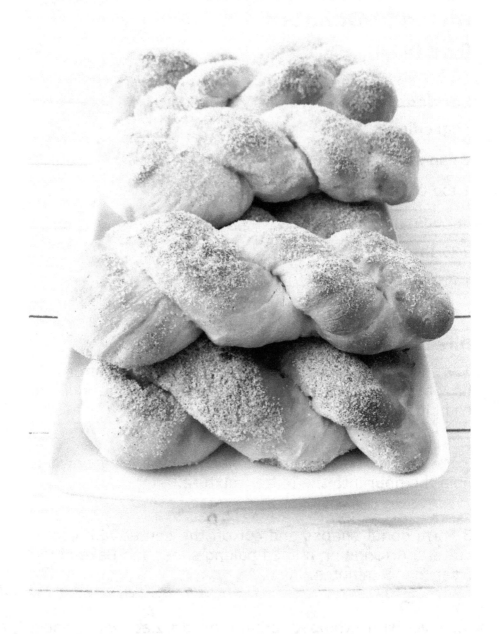

Snickerdoodle Poppers

Cook Time:

30 minutes

Servings:4

Ingredients:

1 box instant vanilla Jell-O mix

1 can Pillsbury Grands Flaky Layers Biscuits

1 ½ cups cinnamon sugar

2 tbsp butter, melted

Directions:

1.Preheat air fryer to 340 F. Unroll the flaky biscuits and cut them into fourths.

2.Roll each ¼ into a ball. Arrange the balls on a paper-lined baking sheet and Bake in the air fryer for 7 minutes or until golden.

3.Prepare the Jell-O following the package's instructions. Using an injector, insert some of the vanilla pudding into each ball.

4.Brush the balls with melted butter and then coat with cinnamon sugar. Enjoy!

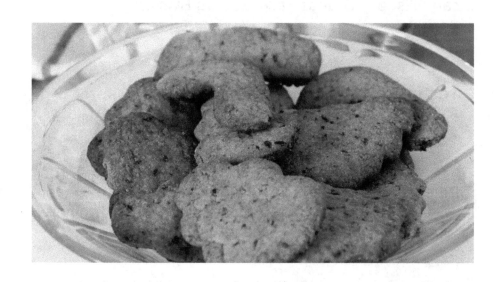

Awesome Chocolate Fudge

Cook Time:

35 minutes

Servings:4/6

Ingredients:

1 cup sugar

1 cup plain flour

1 tbsp honey

¼ cup milk

1 tsp vanilla extract

1 tbsp cocoa powder

2 eggs

½ cup butter, softened

1 orange, juice and zest

Icing:

1 oz butter, melted

4 oz powdered sugar

1 tbsp milk

2 tsp honey

Directions:

1.Preheat air fryer to 350 F. In a bowl, mix sugar, flour, orange zest, and cocoa powder.

2.In another bowl, beat eggs, butter, honey, milk, vanilla, and orange juice until creamy.

3.Combine the two mixtures. Transfer the batter to a greased cake pan and Bake in the air fryer for 23-26 minutes, until set and golden.

4.Remove and let cool. Whisk together all icing ingredients in a bowl. When the cake is chilled, top with the icing, slice, and serve. Enjoy!

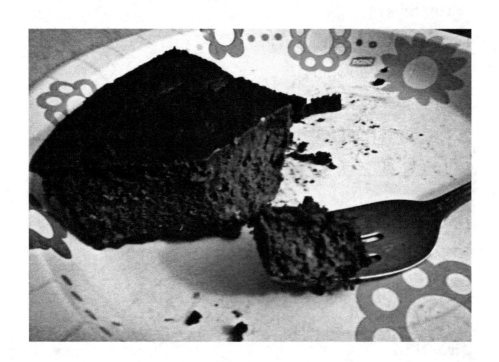

Oat & Walnut Granola

Cook Time:

30 minutes

Servings:4

Ingredients:

¼ cup walnuts, chopped

½ cup oats

3 tbsp canola oil

½ cup maple syrup

2 tbsp muscovado sugar

1 cup fresh blueberries

Directions:

1.Preheat air fryer to 380 F. In a bowl, place oil, maple syrup, muscovado sugar, and vanilla and mix.

2.Coat in the oats. Spread out the mixture on a greased baking tray and Bake for 20-25 minutes.

3.Sprinkle with blueberries and bake for another 3 minutes. Leave to cool before breaking up and storing in a jar. Enjoy!

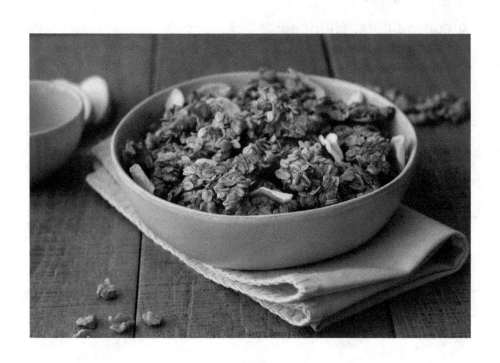

Easy Chocolate Squares

Cook Time:

30 minutes

Servings:2

Ingredients:

1 whole egg, beaten

¼ cup chocolate chips

2 tbsp white sugar

⅓ cup flour

2 tbsp olive oil

¼ cup cocoa powder

Directions:

1.Preheat air fryer to 330 F. In a bowl, mix the egg, sugar, and olive oil until creamy.

2.In another bowl, mix the cocoa powder and flour. Add the flour mixture to the egg mixture and stir until fully incorporated.

3.Pour the mixture into a greased baking dish. Sprinkle chocolate chips on top and Bake in the fryer for 20 minutes. Let cool, slice into squares, and serve. Enjoy!

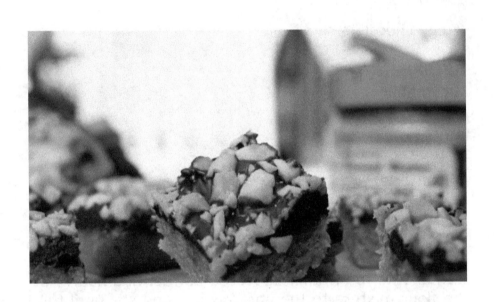

24

Effortless Pecan Pie

Preparation Time:

40 minutes

Cook Time:

30 minutes

Servings:4

Ingredients:

¾ cup maple syrup

2 eggs

¼ tsp ground nutmeg

½ tsp cinnamon

2 tbsp almond butter

2 tbsp brown sugar

½ cup pecans, chopped

1 tbsp butter, melted

1 8-inch pie dough

¾ tsp vanilla extract

Directions:

1.Preheat air fryer to 360 F. Coat the pecans with melted butter. Place them in the frying basket and Bake for 8-10 minutes, shaking once.

2.Place the pie crust into a 7-inch round pie pan and pour the pecans over. Whisk together all the remaining ingredients in a bowl.

3.Spread the maple syrup mixture over the pecans. Set the air fryer to 320 F and Bake the pie for 25 minutes. Serve chilled. Enjoy!

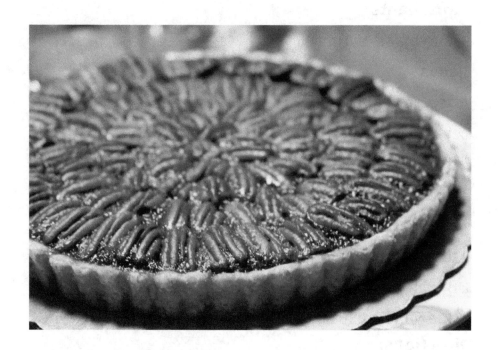

Simple Coffee Cake

Cook Time:

30 minutes

Servings:2

Ingredients:

¼ cup butter

½ tsp instant coffee 1

 tbsp black coffee, brewed

1 egg

¼ cup sugar

¼ cup flour

1 tsp cocoa powder Powdered sugar, for icing

Directions:

1.Preheat air fryer to 320 F. In a bowl, beat sugar and egg until creamy.

2.Mix in cocoa, instant and black coffees; stir in flour. Transfer the batter to a greased baking dish. Bake in the air fryer for 15 minutes.

3.Let cool for at least 1 hour at room temperature. Dust with powdered sugar, slice and serve.

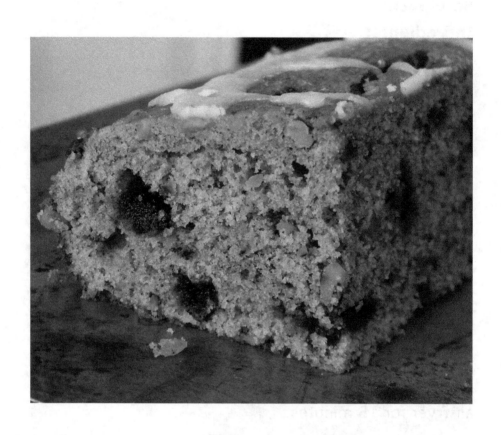

Honey & Cherry Rice

Cook Time:

30 minutes

Servings:4

Ingredients:

1 cup long-grain rice

2 cups milk

½ cup cherries, chopped

3 tbsp honey

1 tsp vanilla extract

1/3 cup heavy cream

Directions:

1.Preheat air fryer to 360 F. In a baking dish, combine all the ingredients, except for the cherries.

2.Place the dish in the air fryer and Bake for 20 minutes. Spoon into glass cups and top with cherries to serve. Enjoy!

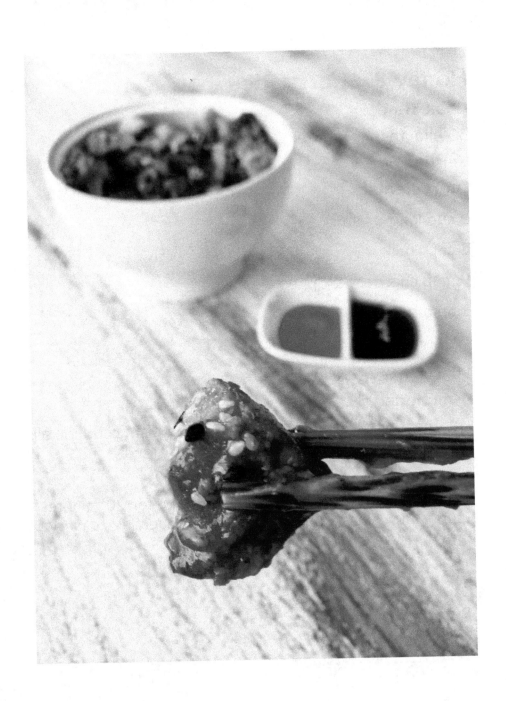

Cheat Apple Pie

Cook Time:

30 minutes

Servings:4

Ingredients:

2 apples, diced

2 tbsp butter, melted

2 tbsp white sugar

1 tbsp brown sugar

1 tsp cinnamon

1 egg, beaten

2 large puff pastry sheets

¼ tsp salt

DIRECTIONS:

1.Whisk white sugar, brown sugar, cinnamon, salt, and butter. Place the apples in a greased baking dish and coat them with the mixture.

2.Place the dish in the air fryer and Bake for 10 minutes at 350 F. Meanwhile, roll out the pastry on a floured flat surface and cut each sheet into 6 equal pieces. Divide the apple filling between the pieces.

3.Brush the edges of the pastry squares with the egg. Fold the squares and seal the edges with a fork.

4.Place on a lined baking sheet and Bake in the fryer at 350 F for 8 minutes. Flip over, increase the heat to 320 F, and cook for 2 more minutes. Serve chilled. Enjoy!

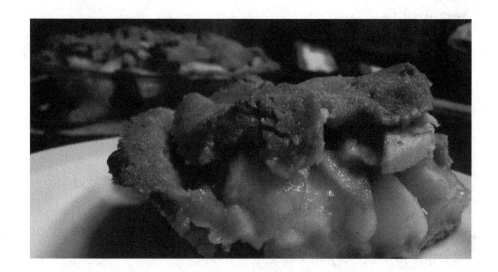

Chocolate Mug Cake

Cook Time:

10 minutes

Servings:2

Ingredients:

1/2 cup self-rising flour

6 tablespoons brown sugar

5 tablespoons coconut milk

4 tablespoons coconut oil

4 tablespoons unsweetened cocoa powder

2 eggs

A pinch of grated nutmeg

A pinch of salt

Directions:

1.Mix all the ingredients together; divide the batter between two mugs.

2.Place the mugs in the Air Fryer cooking basket and cook at 390 degrees F for about 10 minutes. Enjoy!

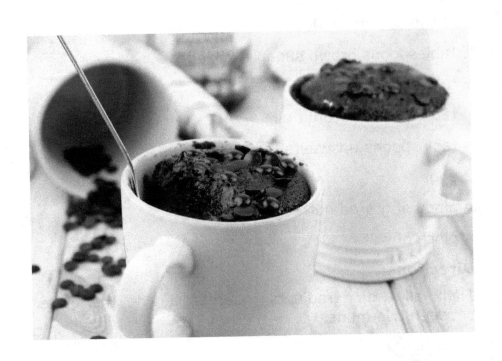

Old-Fashioned Baked Pears

Cook Time:

10 minutes

Servings:2

Ingredients:

2 large pears, halved and cored

1 teaspoon lemon juice

2 teaspoons coconut oil

1/2 cup rolled oats

1/4 cup walnuts, chopped

1/4 cup brown sugar

1 teaspoon apple pie spice mix

Directions:

1.Drizzle the pear halves with lemon juice and coconut oil. In a mixing bowl, thoroughly combine the rolled oats, walnuts, brown sugar and apple pie spice mix.

2.Cook in the preheated Air Fryer at 360 degrees for 8 minutes, checking them halfway through the cooking time. Dust with powdered sugar if desired. Enjoy!

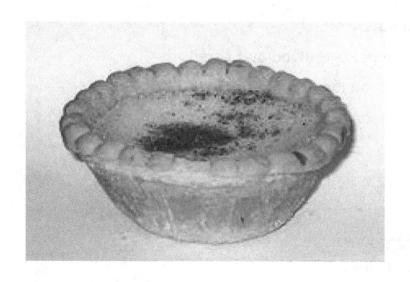

Easy Monkey Rolls

Cook Time:

25 minutes

Servings:4

Ingredients:

8 ounces refrigerated buttermilk biscuit dough

1/2 cup brown sugar

4 ounces butter, melted

1/4 teaspoon grated nutmeg

1/2 teaspoon ground cinnamon

1/4 teaspoon ground cardamom

Directions:

1.Spritz 4 standard-size muffin cups with a nonstick spray. Thoroughly combine the brown sugar with the melted butter, nutmeg, cinnamon and cardamom.

2.Spoon the butter mixture into muffins cups. Separate the dough into biscuits and divide your biscuits between muffin cups.

3.Bake the Monkey rolls at 340 degrees F for about 15 minutes or until golden brown. Turn upside down just before serving. Enjoy!

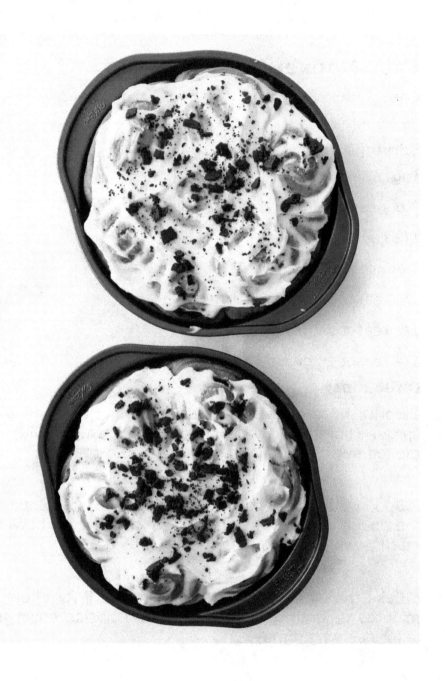

Chocolate Apple Chips

Cook Time:

15 minutes

Servings:6

Ingredients:

1 large Pink Lady apple, cored and sliced

1 tablespoon light brown sugar

A pinch of kosher salt

2 tablespoons lemon juice

2 teaspoons cocoa powder

Directions:

1.Toss the apple slices with the other ingredients. Bake at 350 degrees F for 5 minutes; shake the basket to ensure even cooking and continue to cook an additional 5 minutes. Enjoy!

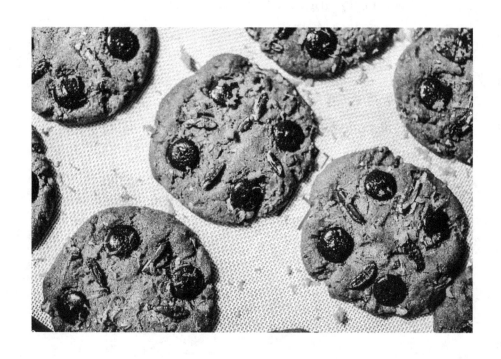

Chocolate Biscuit Sandwich Cookies

Cook Time:

20 minutes

Servings:10

Ingredients:

2 ½ cups self-rising flour

4 ounces brown sugar

1 ounce honey

5 ounces butter, softened

1 egg, beaten

1 teaspoon vanilla essence

4 ounces double cream

3 ounces dark chocolate

1 teaspoon cardamom seeds, finely crushed

Directions:

1.Start by preheating your Air Fryer to 350 degrees F. In a mixing bowl, thoroughly combine the flour, brown sugar, honey, and butter.

2.Mix until your mixture resembles breadcrumbs. Gradually, add the egg and vanilla essence.

3.Shape your dough into small balls and place in the parchment-lined Air Fryer basket. Bake in the preheated Air Fryer for 10 minutes.

4.Rotate the pan and bake for another 5 minutes. Transfer the freshly baked cookies to a cooling rack.

5.As the biscuits are cooling, melt the double cream and dark chocolate in an air-fryer safe bowl at 350 degrees F.

6.Add the cardamom seeds and stir well. Spread the filling over the cooled biscuits and sandwich together. Enjoy!

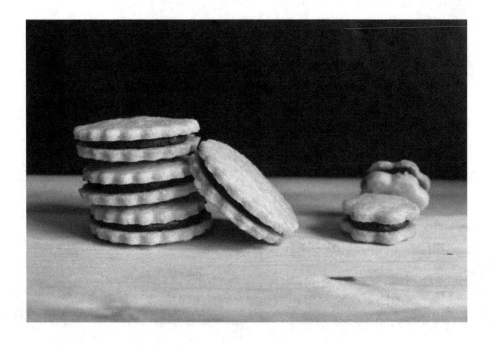

Rustic Baked Apples

Cook Time:

25 minutes

Servings:4

Ingredients:

4 Gala apples

1/4 cup rolled oats

1/4 cup sugar

2 tablespoons honey

1/3 cup walnuts, chopped

1 teaspoon cinnamon powder

1/2 teaspoon ground cardamom

1/2 teaspoon ground cloves

2/3 cup water

Directions:

1.Use a paring knife to remove the stem and seeds from the apples, making deep holes.

2.In a mixing bowl, combine together the rolled oats, sugar, honey, walnuts, cinnamon, cardamom, and cloves. Pour the water into an Air Fryer safe dish.

3.Place the apples in the dish. Bake at 340 degrees F for 17 minutes. Serve at room temperature. Enjoy!

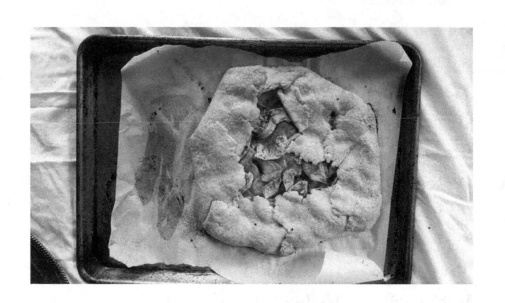

Chocolate Birthday Cake

Cook Time:

35 minutes

Servings:6

Ingredients:

2 eggs, beaten

2/3 cup sour cream

1 cup flour

1/2 cup sugar

1/4 cup honey

1/3 cup coconut oil, softened

1/4 cup cocoa powder

2 tablespoons chocolate chips

1 ½ teaspoons baking powder

1 teaspoon vanilla extract

1/2 teaspoon pure rum extract

Chocolate Frosting:

1/2 cup butter, softened

1/4 cup cocoa powder

2 cups powdered sugar

2 tablespoons milk

Directions:

1.Mix all ingredients for the chocolate cake with a hand mixer on low speed. Scrape the batter into a cake pan. Bake at 330 degrees F for 25 to 30 minutes.

2.Transfer the cake to a wire rack Meanwhile, whip the butter and cocoa until smooth. Stir in the powdered sugar.

3.Slowly and gradually, pour in the milk until your frosting reaches desired consistency. Whip until smooth and fluffy; then, frost the cooled cake.

4.Place in your refrigerator for a couple of hours. Serve well chilled. Enjoy!

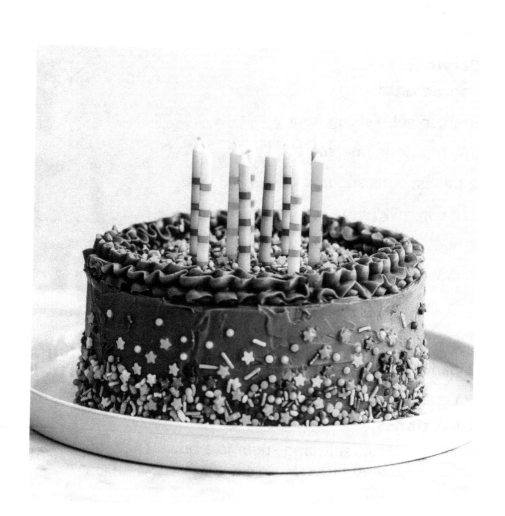

Greek -Style Griddle Cakes

Cook Time:

25 minutes

Servings:4

Ingredients:

3/4 cup self-raising flour

1/4 teaspoon fine sea salt

2 tablespoons sugar

1/2 cup milk

2 eggs, lightly beaten

1 tablespoon butter

Topping:

1 cup Greek-style yogurt

1 banana, mashed

2 tablespoons honey

Directions:

1.Mix the flour, salt, and sugar in a bowl. Then, stir in the milk, eggs, and butter.

2.Mix until smooth and uniform. Drop tablespoons of the batter into the Air Fryer pan.

3.Cook at 300 degrees F for 4 to 5 minutes or until bubbles form on top of the griddle cakes. Repeat with the remaining batter.

4.Meanwhile, mix all ingredients for the topping. Place in your refrigerator until ready to serve. Serve the griddle cakes with the chilled topping. Enjoy!

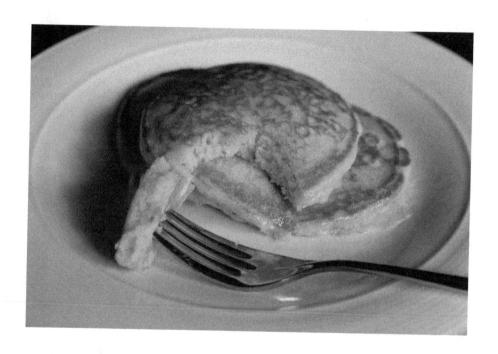

Classic Butter Cake

Cook Time:

35 minutes

Servings:8

Ingredients:

1 stick butter, at room temperature

1 cup sugar

2 eggs

1 cup all-purpose flour

1 teaspoon baking powder

1/2 teaspoon baking soda

1/4 teaspoon salt

A pinch of freshly grated nutmeg

A pinch of ground star anise

1/4 cup buttermilk

1 teaspoon vanilla essence

Directions:

1.Begin by preheating your Air Fryer to 320 degrees F. Spritz the bottom and sides of a baking pan with cooking spray.

2.Beat the butter and sugar with a hand mixer until creamy. Then, fold in the eggs, one at a time, and mix well until fluffy.

3.Stir in the flour along with the remaining ingredients. Mix to combine well.

4.Scrape the batter into the prepared baking pan. Bake for 15 minutes; rotate the pan and bake an additional 15 minutes, until the top of the cake springs back when gently pressed with your fingers. Enjoy!

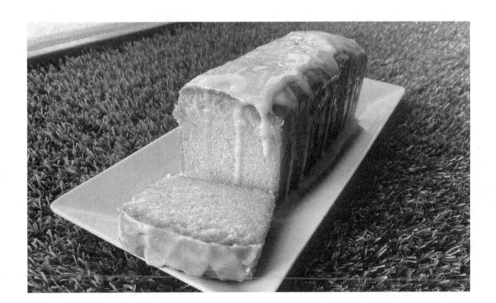

White Chocolate Rum Molten Cake

Cook Time:

20 minutes

Servings:4

Ingredients:

2 ½ ounces butter, at room temperature

3 ounces white chocolate

2 eggs, beaten

1/2 cup powdered sugar

1/3 cup self-rising flour

1 teaspoon rum extract

1 teaspoon vanilla extract

Directions:

1.Begin by preheating your Air Fryer to 370 degrees F. Spritz the sides and bottom of four ramekins with cooking spray.

2.Melt the butter and white chocolate in a microwave-safe bowl.

3.Mix the eggs and sugar until frothy. Pour the butter/chocolate mixture into the egg mixture. Stir in the flour, rum extract, and vanilla extract.

4.Mix until everything is well incorporated. Scrape the batter into the prepared ramekins.

5.Bake in the preheated Air Fryer for 9 to 11 minutes. Let stand for 2 to 3 minutes. Invert on a plate while warm and serve. Enjoy!

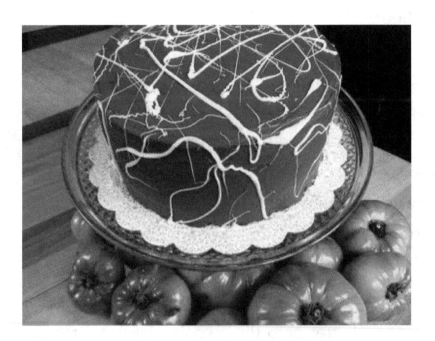

Old-Fashioned Pinch-Me Cake with Walnuts

Cook Time:

20 minutes

Servings:4

Ingredients:

1 10-ounces can crescent rolls

1/2 stick butter

1/2 cup caster sugar

1 teaspoon pumpkin pie spice blend

1 tablespoon dark rum

1/2 cup walnuts, chopped

Directions:

1.Start by preheating your Air Fryer to 350 degrees F. Roll out the crescent rolls.

2.Spread the butter onto the crescent rolls; scatter the sugar, spices and walnuts over the rolls.

3.Drizzle with rum and roll them up. Using your fingertips, gently press them to seal the edges.

4.Bake your cake for about 13 minutes or until the top is golden brown. Enjoy!

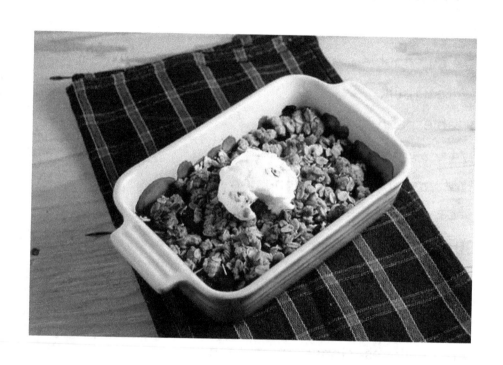

Crunchy French Toast Sticks

Cook Time:

10 minutes

Servings:3

Ingredients:

1 egg

1/4 cup double cream

1/4 cup milk

1 tablespoon brown sugar

1/4 teaspoon ground cloves

1/4 teaspoon ground cinnamon

1/4 vanilla paste

3thick slices of brioche bread, cut into thirds

1 cup crispy rice cereal

Directions:

1.Thoroughly combine the egg, cream, milk, sugar, ground cloves, cinnamon and vanilla.

2.Dip each piece of bread into the cream mixture and then, press gently into the cereal, pressing to coat all sides.

3.Arrange the pieces of bread in the Air Fryer cooking basket and cook them at 380 degrees F for 2 minutes;

flip and cook on the other side for 2 to 3 minutes longer. Enjoy!

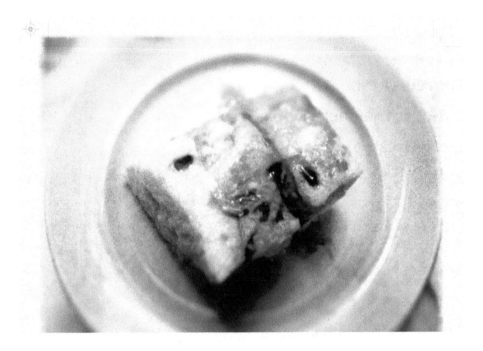

Summer Fruit Pie

Cook Time:

35 minutes

Servings:4

Ingredients:

2 8-ounce refrigerated pie crusts

2 cups fresh blackberries

1/4 cup caster sugar

2 teaspoons cornstarch

A pinch of sea salt

1/4 teaspoon ground nutmeg

1/4 teaspoon ground cinnamon

1/4 teaspoon vanilla extract

Directions:

1.Start by preheating your Air Fryer to 350 degrees F. Place the pie crust in a lightly greased pie plate.

2.In a bowl, combine the fresh blackberries with caster sugar, cornstarch, salt, nutmeg, cinnamon and vanilla extract.

3.Spoon the blackberry filling into the prepared pie crust. Top the blackberry filling with second crust and cut slits in pastry.

4.Bake your pie in the preheated Air Fryer for 35 minutes or until the top is golden brown. Enjoy!

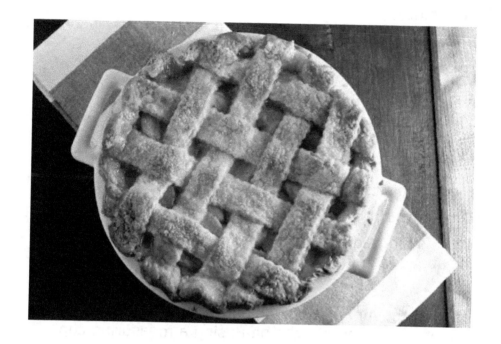

Chocolate Chip Banana Crepes

Cook Time:

30 minutes

Servings:2

Ingredients:

1 small ripe banana

1/8 teaspoon baking powder

1/4 cup chocolate chips

1 egg, whisked

Directions:

1.Mix all ingredients until creamy and fluffy. Let it stand for about 20 minutes.

2.Spritz the Air Fryer baking pan with cooking spray. Pour 1/2 of the batter into the pan using a measuring cup.

3.Cook at 230 degrees F for 4 to 5 minutes or until golden brown. Repeat with another crepe. Enjoy!!

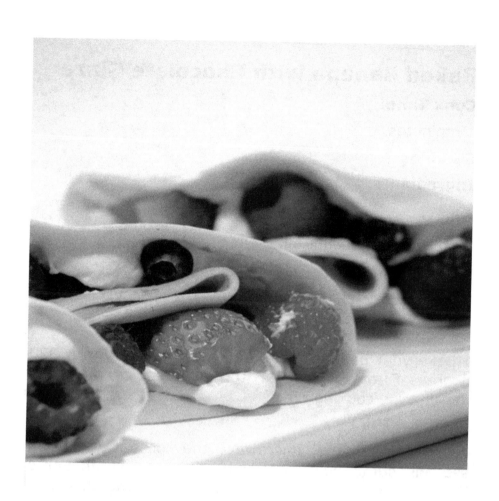

Baked Banana with Chocolate Glaze

Cook Time:

15 minutes

Servings:2

Ingredients:

2 bananas, peeled and cut in half lengthwise

1 tablespoon coconut oil, melted

1 tablespoon cocoa powder

1 tablespoon agave syrup

Directions:

1.Bake your bananas in the preheated Air Fryer at 370 degrees F for 12 minutes, turning them over halfway through the cooking time.

2.In the meantime, microwave the coconut oil for 30 seconds; stir in the cocoa powder and agave syrup. Serve the baked bananas with a few drizzles of the chocolate glaze. Enjoy!

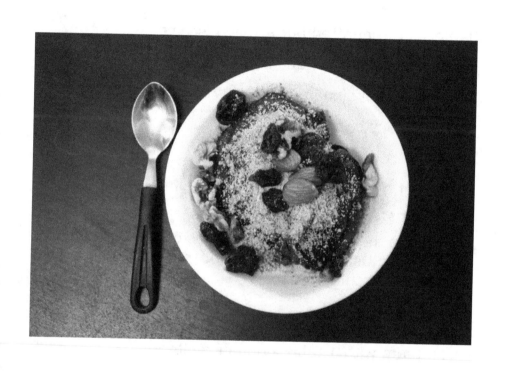

Old-Fashioned Donuts

Cook Time:

15 minutes

Servings:4

Ingredients:

8 ounces refrigerated buttermilk biscuits

2 tablespoons butter, unsalted and melted

1/2 tablespoon cinnamon

4 tablespoons caster sugar

A pinch of salt

A pinch of grated nutmeg

Directions:

1.Separate the biscuits and cut holes out of the center of each biscuit using a 1-inch round biscuit cutter; place them on a parchment paper.

2.Lower your biscuits into the Air Fryer cooking basket. Brush them with 1 tablespoon of melted butter.

3.Air fry your biscuits at 340 degrees F for about 8 minutes or until golden brown, flipping them halfway through the cooking time.

4.Meanwhile, mix the sugar with cinnamon, salt and nutmeg. Brush your donuts with remaining 1 tablespoon of melted butter; roll them in the cinnamon-sugar and serve. Enjoy!

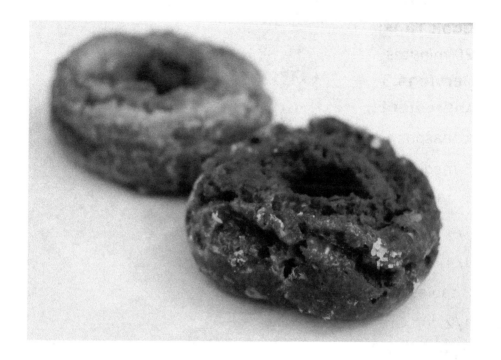

Greek Roasted Figs with Yiaourti me Meli

Cook Time:

20 minutes

Servings:3

Ingredients:

1 teaspoon coconut oil, melted

6 medium-sized figs

1/4 teaspoon ground cardamom

1/4 teaspoon ground cloves

1/4 teaspoon ground cinnamon

3 tablespoon honey

1/2 cup Greek yogurt

Directions:

1.Drizzle the melted coconut oil all over your figs. Sprinkle cardamom, cloves and cinnamon over your figs.

2.Roast your figs in the preheated Air Fryer at 330 degrees F for 15 to 16 minutes, shaking the basket occasionally to promote even cooking.

3.In the meantime, thoroughly combine the honey with the Greek yogurt to make the yiaourti me meli.

4.Divide the roasted figs between 3 serving bowls and serve with a dollop of yiaourti me meli. Enjoy!

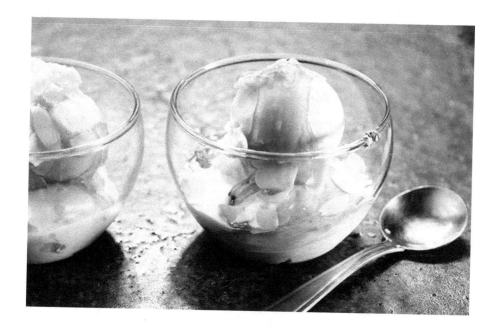

Banana Chips with Chocolate Glaze

Cook Time:

20minutes

Servings:3

Ingredients:

2 banana, cut into slices

1/4 teaspoon lemon zest

1 tablespoon agave syrup

1 tablespoon cocoa powder

1 tablespoon coconut oil, melted

Directions:

1.Toss the bananas with the lemon zest and agave syrup. Transfer your bananas to the parchment-lined cooking basket.

2.Bake in the preheated Air Fryer at 370 degrees F for 12 minutes, turning them over halfway through the cooking time.

3.In the meantime, melt the coconut oil in your microwave; add the cocoa powder and whisk to combine well.

4.Serve the baked banana chips with a few drizzles of the chocolate glaze. Enjoy!

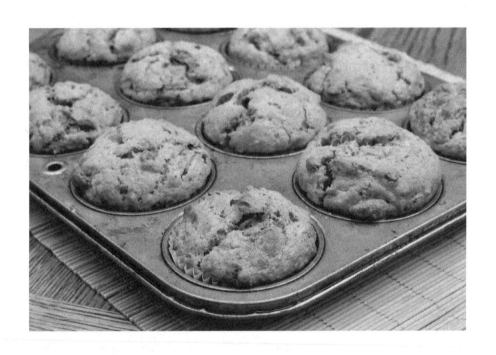

Cinnamon and Sugar Sweet Potato Fries

Cook Time:

30 minutes

Servings: 2

Ingredients:

1 large sweet potato, peeled and sliced into sticks

1 teaspoon ghee

1 tablespoon cornstarch

1/4 teaspoon ground cardamom

1/4 cup sugar

1 tablespoon ground cinnamon

Directions:

1.Toss the sweet potato sticks with the melted ghee and cornstarch.

2.Cook in the preheated Air Fryer at 380 degrees F for 20 minutes, shaking the basket halfway through the cooking time.

3.Sprinkle the cardamom, sugar, and cinnamon all over the sweet potato fries and serve. Enjoy!

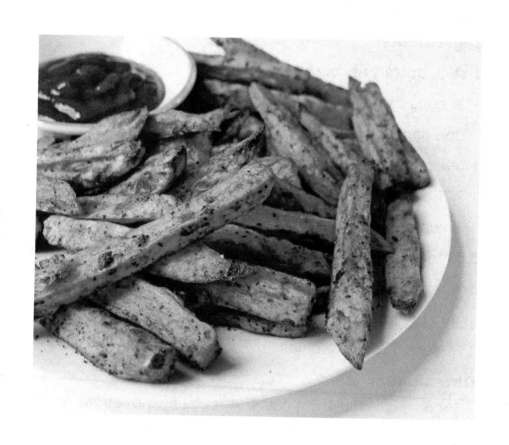

Sunday Banana Chocolate Cookies

Cook Time:

30 minutes

Servings:8

Ingredients:

1 stick butter, at room temperature

1 ¼ cups caster sugar

2 ripe bananas, mashed

1 teaspoon vanilla paste

1 2/3 cups all-purpose flour

1/3 cup cocoa powder

1 ½ teaspoons baking powder

1/4 teaspoon ground cinnamon

1/4 teaspoon crystallized ginger

1 ½ cups chocolate chips

Directions:

1.In a mixing dish, beat the butter and sugar until creamy and uniform. Stir in the mashed bananas and vanilla.

2.In another mixing dish, thoroughly combine the flour, cocoa powder, baking powder, cinnamon, and crystallized ginger.

3.Add the flour mixture to the banana mixture; mix to combine well.

4.Afterwards, fold in the chocolate chips. Drop by large spoonfuls onto a parchment-lined Air Fryer basket.

5.Bake at 365 degrees F for 11 minutes or until golden brown on the top. enjoy!

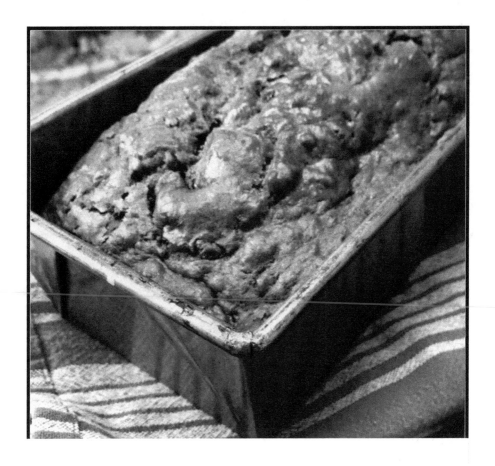

French Sour Cherry Clafoutis

Cook Time:

30 minutes + cooling time

Servings:4

Ingredients:

½ lb sour cherries, pitted

½ cup all-purpose flour

¼ tsp salt

2 tbsp sugar

2 eggs + 2 yolks

1 tsp vanilla extract

1 tbsp lemon zest

2 tbsp butter, melted

1 ¼ cups milk Icing sugar to dust

Directions:

1.Preheat air fryer to 380 F. In a bowl, mix the flour, sugar, and salt.

2.Whisk in the eggs, egg yolks, vanilla extract, lemon zest, and melted butter until creamy. Gradually, add in the milk and stir until bubbly.

3.Spread the sour cherries on a greased baking dish and pour over the batter.

4.Bake in the air fryer for 25-30 minutes until a lovely golden crust is formed. Dust the top with icing sugar and serve warm.Enjoy!

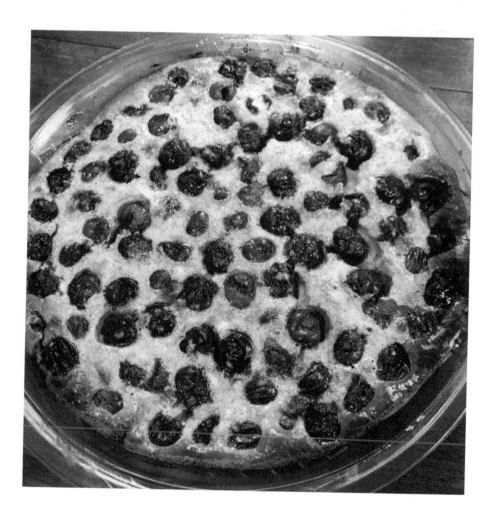

Apple Caramel Relish

Cook Time:

30 minutes

Serving:4

Ingredients:

1 vanilla box cake mix

2 apples, peeled, sliced

3 oz butter, melted

½ cup brown sugar

1 tsp cinnamon

½ cup flour

1 cup caramel sauce

Directions:

1.Line a cake tin with baking paper. In a bowl, mix butter, sugar, cinnamon, and flour until you obtain a crumbly texture.

2.Prepare the cake mix according to the instructions no baking. Pour the obtained batter into the tin and arrange the apple slices on top.

3.Spoon the caramel over the apples and pour the crumbly flour mixture over the sauce.

4.Bake in the preheated air fryer for 18-20 minutes at 360 F. Check halfway through to avoid overcooking. Serve chilled. Enjoy!

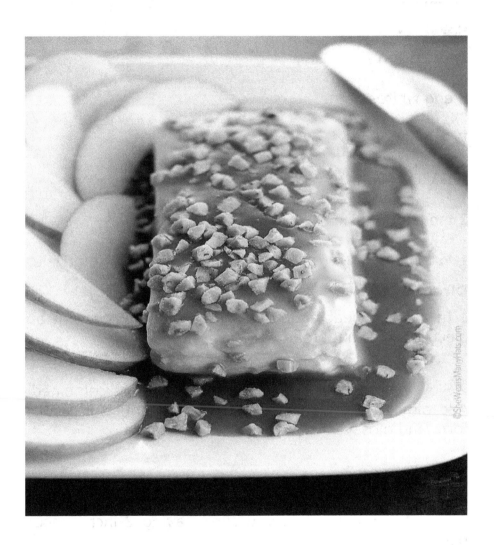

Madrid-Style Almond Meringues

Cook Time:

30 minutes

Servings:4

Ingredients:

8 egg whites

½ tsp almond extract

1 ⅓ cups sugar

2 tsp lemon juice

1 ½ tsp vanilla extract Melted dark chocolate, to drizzle

Directions:

1.In a bowl, beat egg whites and lemon juice with an electric mixer until foamy.

2.Slowly beat in the sugar until thoroughly combined. Add almond and vanilla extracts. Beat until stiff peaks form and glossy.

3.Line a baking tray with parchment paper. Fill a piping bag with the meringue mixture and pipe as many mounds on the baking sheet as you can, leaving 2-inch spaces between each mound.

4.Place the baking tray in the frying basket and Bake at 250 F for 5 minutes.

5.Reduce the temperature to 220 F and bake for 15 more minutes.

6.Then, reduce the temperature to 190 F and cook for 13-15 more minutes. Let the meringues cool. Drizzle with dark chocolate and serve. Enjoy!

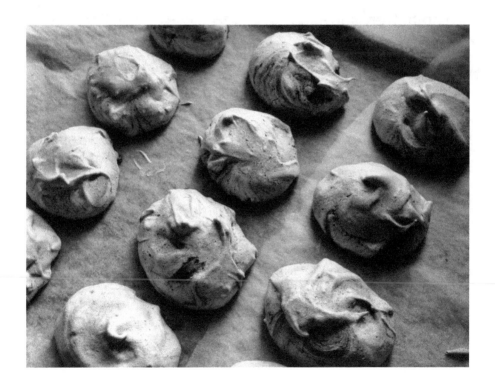

Dark Rum Pear Pie

Cook Time:

30 minutes

Servings:4

Ingredients:

1 cup flour

5 tbsp sugar

3 tbsp butter, softened

1 tbsp dark spiced rum

2 pears, sliced

Directions:

1.Preheat air fryer to 370 F. In a bowl, place 3 tbsp of the sugar, butter, and flour and mix to form a batter.

2.Roll out the butter on a floured surface and transfer to the greased baking dish.

3.Arrange the pears slices on top and sprinkle with sugar and dark rum. Bake in the air fryer for 20 minutes. Serve cooled. Enjoy!

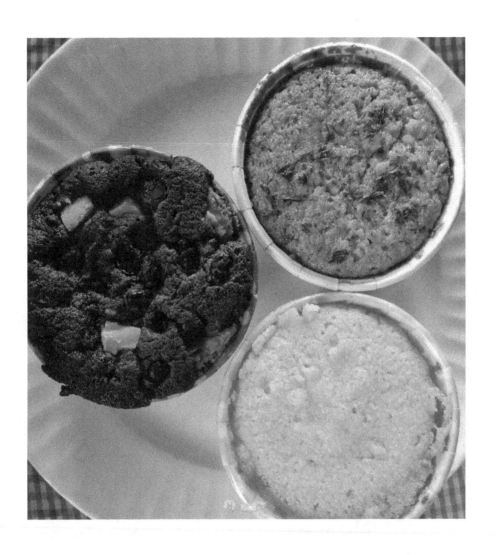

Chocolate Soufflé

Cook Time:

30 minutes

Servings:2

Ingredients:

2 eggs, whites and yolks separated

¼ cup butter, melted

2 tbsp flour

3 tbsp sugar

3 oz chocolate, melted

½ tsp vanilla extract

Directions:

1.Preheat air fryer to 320 F. In a bowl, beat the yolks along with sugar and vanilla extract until creamy. Stir in butter, chocolate, and flour.

2.In another bowl, whisk the whites until stiff peak forms. Working in batches, gently combine the egg whites with the chocolate mixture.

3.Divide the batter between two greased ramekins. Bake in the air fryer for 14 minutes. Serve warm or at room temperature. Enjoy!

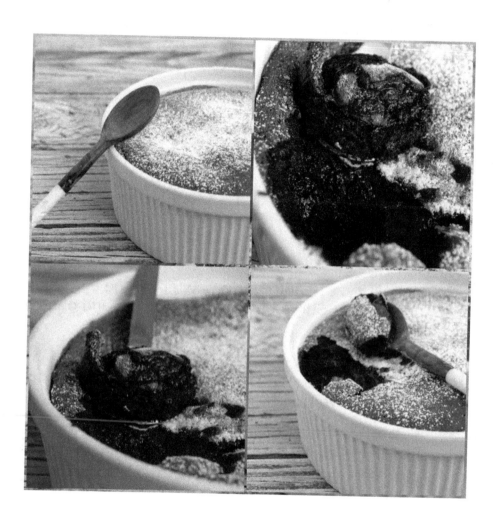

Molten Lava Cake

Cook Time:

30 minutes

Servings:4

Ingredients:

2 tbsp butter, melted

3 ½ tbsp sugar

1 ½ tbsp self-rising flour

3 ½ oz dark chocolate, melted

2 eggs

Directions:

1.Preheat air fryer to 360 F. In a bowl, beat the eggs and sugar until frothy. Stir in butter and chocolate and gently fold in the flour.

2.Divide the mixture between 4 greased ramekins and Bake in the air fryer for 18 minutes.

3.Let cool for a few minutes before inverting the lava cakes onto serving plates. Enjoy!

Spanish Churros con Chocolate

Cook Time:

30 minutes

Servings:4

Ingredients:

1 tsp vanilla extract

¼ cup butter

½ cup water

1 pinch of salt

½ cup all-purpose flour

2 eggs

¼ cup white sugar

½ tsp ground cinnamon

4 oz dark chocolate chips

¼ cup milk

Directions:

1.In a skillet over medium heat, pour water, sugar, butter, and a pinch of salt; bring to a boil.

2.Stir in the flour until the mixture is thick, about 3 minutes. Remove to a bowl, mix in vanilla, and let cool slightly.

3.Preheat air fryer to 360 F. Gently stir in the eggs, one at a time, until glossy and smooth.

4.Place the dough in a piping bag and grease the frying basket with cooking spray.

5.Pipe in the batter into strips. Place in the air fryer and Air Fryer for 8-10 minutes until golden.

6.Mix the chocolate with cinnamon in a heatproof bowl and microwave for 60-90 seconds until the chocolate is melted. Stir in milk until smooth.

7.Serve the churros with hot chocolate. Enjoy!

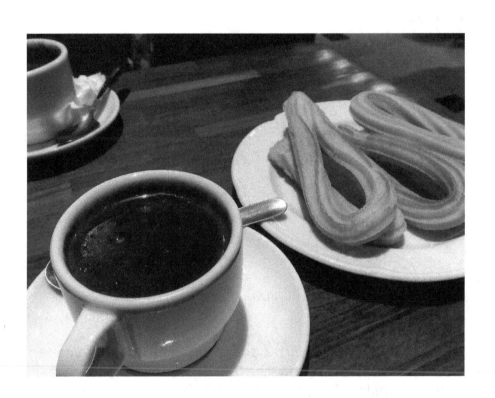

Vanilla & Chocolate Brownies

Cook Time:

30 minutes

Servings:4

Ingredients:

6 oz dark chocolate

6 oz butter

¾ cup white sugar

3 eggs

2 tsp vanilla extract

¾ cup flour

¼ cup cocoa powder

1 cup walnuts, chopped

1 cup white chocolate chips

Directions:

1.Line a baking dish with baking paper. Place a saucepan over low heat and melt the dark chocolate and butter, stirring constantly until a smooth mixture is obtained; let cool slightly.

2.In a bowl, whisk eggs, sugar, and vanilla. Sift flour and cocoa and stir in the egg mixture to combine.

3.Sprinkle the walnuts over and add white chocolate chips and melted dark chocolate into the batter; stir well.

4.Spread the batter onto the dish and Bake in the preheated air fryer for 20 minutes at 340 F. Enjoy!

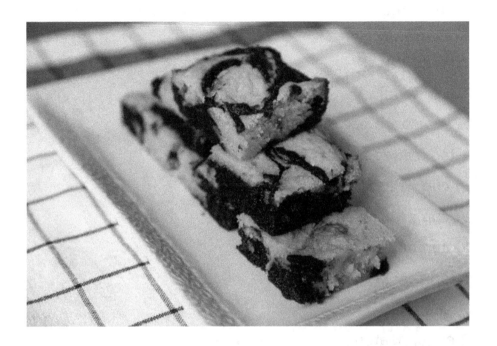

Chocolate & Raspberry Cake

Cook Time:

30 minutes

Servings:6

Ingredients:

1 cup flour

⅓ cup cocoa powder

1 tsp baking powder

½ cup white sugar

¼ cup brown sugar

½ cup butter, melted

1 tsp vanilla extract

⅔ cup milk

2 eggs, beaten

1 cup raspberries

1 cup chocolate chips

Directions:

1.Line a cake tin with baking paper. In a bowl, sift flour, cocoa powder, and baking powder.

2.In another bowl, whisk butter, white and brown sugar, vanilla, and milk until creamy.

3.Mix in the eggs. Pour the wet ingredients into the dry ones, and fold to combine.

4.Add in the raspberries and chocolate chips. Pour the batter into the lined tin and Bake in the air fryer for 20 minutes at 350 F. Serve cooled. Enjoy!

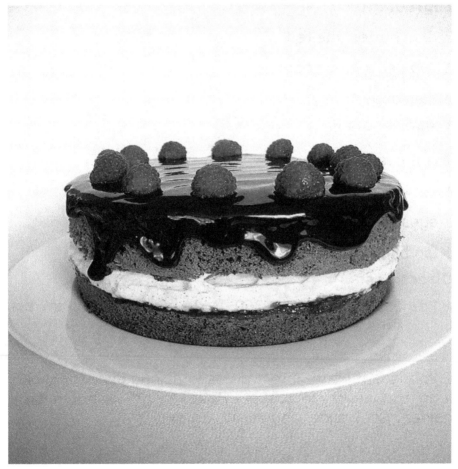

Peach Almond Flour Cake

Cook Time:

30 minutes

Servings:4

Ingredients:

3 tbsp butter, melted

1 cup peaches, chopped

3 tbsp sugar

1 cup almond flour

1 cup heavy cream

1 tsp vanilla extract

2 eggs, whisked

1 tsp baking soda

Directions:

1.Preheat air fryer to 360 F. In a bowl, mix all the ingredients and stir well.

2.Pour the mixture into a greased baking dish and insert it in the air fryer basket. Bake for 25 minutes until golden. Cool, slice, and serve. Enjoy!

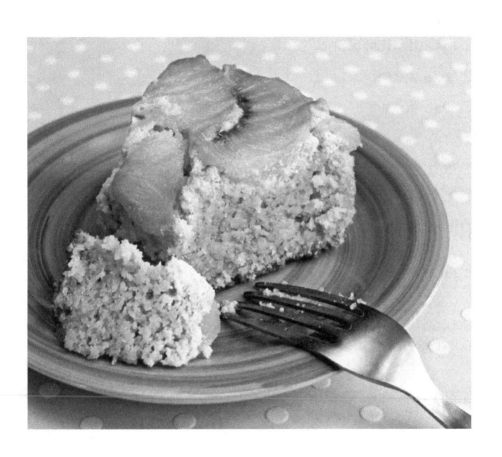

Mom's Lemon Curd

Cook Time:

30 minutes

Servings: 2

Ingredients:

3 tbsp butter

3 tbsp sugar

1 egg

1 egg yolk

¾ lemon, juiced

Directions:

1. Add sugar and butter to a medium-size ramekin and beat evenly.

2. Slowly whisk in egg and egg yolk until fresh yellow color is obtained.

3. Mix in the lemon juice. Place the ramekin in the preheated air fryer and Bake at 220 F for 6 minutes.

4. Increase the temperature to 320 F and cook for 13-15 minutes. Remove the ramekin and use a spoon to check for any lumps. Serve chilled. Enjoy!

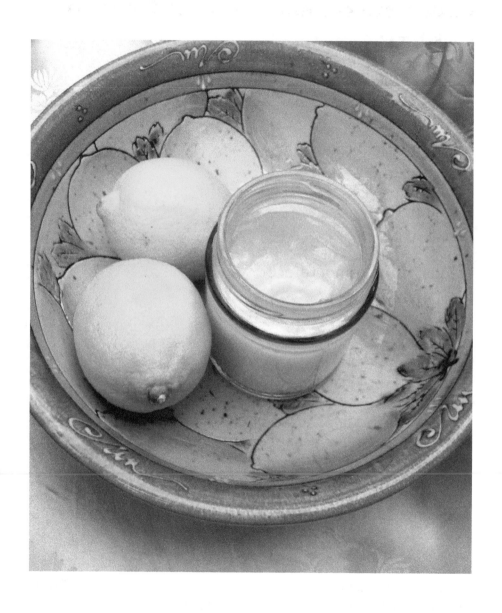

Chocolate & Peanut Butter Fondants

Cook Time:

30 minutes

Servings:4

Ingredients:

¾ cup dark chocolate

½ cup peanut butter, crunchy

2 tbsp butter

½ cup sugar, divided

4 eggs, room temperature

⅛ cup flour, sieved

1 tsp salt

¼ cup water

Directions:

1.Make the praline by adding ¼ cup of sugar, 1 tsp of salt, and water in a saucepan over low heat. Stir and bring to a boil.

2.Simmer until the mixture reduces by half, about 5 minutes.

3.Spread on a baking tray to let cool and harden. Then break into pieces and set aside the pralines. Preheat air fryer to 300 F.

4.Place a pot of water over medium heat and place a heatproof bowl on top.

5.Add in chocolate, butter, and peanut butter. Stir continuously until fully melted, combined, and smooth. Remove the bowl, and let cool slightly.

6.Whisk in the eggs, add flour and remaining sugar; mix well. Grease 4 small loaf pans with cooking spray and divide the chocolate mixture between them.

7.Place them in the air fryer and Bake for 7 minutes. Remove and serve with a piece of praline. Enjoy!

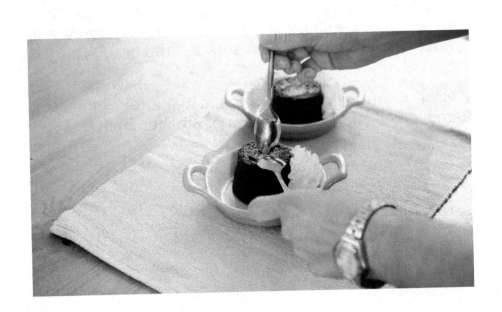

Easy Lemony Cheesecake

Cook Time:

40 minutes

Servings:8

Ingredients:

8 oz graham crackers, crushed

4 oz butter, melted

16 oz plain cream cheese

3 eggs 3 tbsp sugar

1 tbsp vanilla extract

Zest of 2 lemons

DIRECTIONS

1.Line a cake tin that fits in your air fryer with baking paper.

2.Mix together the crackers and butter and press at the bottom of the tin. In a bowl, add cream cheese, eggs, sugar, vanilla, and lemon zest and beat with a hand mixer until well combined and smooth.

3.Pour the mixture on top of the cracker's base. Bake in the air fryer for 20 minutes at 350 F.

4.Regularly check to ensure it's set but still a bit wobbly. Let cool, then refrigerate overnight. Serve at room temperature or chilled. Enjoy!

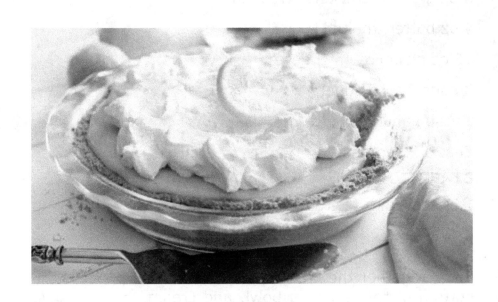

Soft Buttermilk Biscuits

Cook Time:

30 minutes

Servings:10

Ingredients:

1 cup all-purpose flour

¾ tsp salt

½ tsp baking powder

4 tbsp butter, cubed

1 tsp sugar

¾ cup buttermilk

Directions:

1.Preheat air fryer to 360 F. In a bowl, whisk flour, baking powder, sugar, and salt until well combined.

2.Add in butter and rub it into the flour mixture until crumbed.

3.Stir in the buttermilk until a dough is formed. Flour a flat and dry surface and roll out the dough until half-inch thick.

4.Cut out 10 rounds with a small cookie cutter. Arrange the biscuits on a greased baking tray.

5.Working in batches, Bake in the air fryer for 16-18 minutes. Let cool for a few minutes before serving. Enjoy!

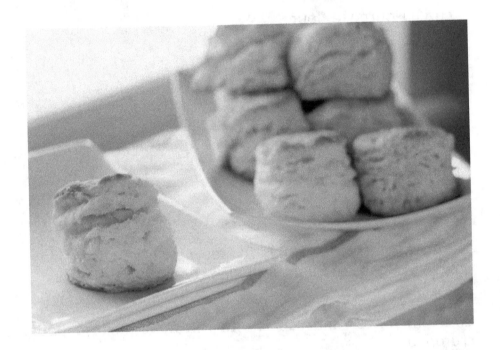

White Chocolate Cookies

Cook Time:

30 minutes

Servings:4

Ingredients:

1 cup self-rising flour

4 tbsp brown sugar

1 egg

2 oz white chocolate chips

1 tbsp honey

1 ½ tbsp milk

1 tsp baking soda

½ cup butter, softened

Directions:

1.Preheat air fryer to 350 F. In a bowl, beat butter and sugar until fluffy.

2.Mix in honey, egg, and milk. In a separate bowl, mix flour and baking soda and gradually add to the butter while stirring constantly.

3.Gently fold in the chocolate cookies. Drop spoonfuls of the mixture onto a greased cookie sheet and press down slightly to flatten.

4.Bake in the air fryer for 18 minutes. Remove to a wire rack to cool completely before serving. Enjoy!

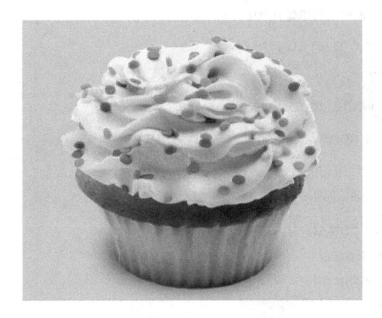

Pineapple Cake

Cook Time:

30 minutes

Servings:4

Ingredients:

2 oz dark chocolate, grated

8 oz self-rising flour

4 oz butter

7 oz pineapple chunks

½ cup pineapple juice

1 egg

2 tbsp milk

½ cup sugar

Directions:

1.Preheat air fryer to 350 F. Place the butter and flour into a bowl and rub the mixture with your fingers until crumbed.

2.Stir in pineapple chunks, sugar, chocolate, and pineapple juice. Beat eggs and milk separately and add to the batter.

3.Transfer the batter to a greased cake pan and Bake in the air fryer for 25 minutes. Let cool for a few minutes before serving. Enjoy!

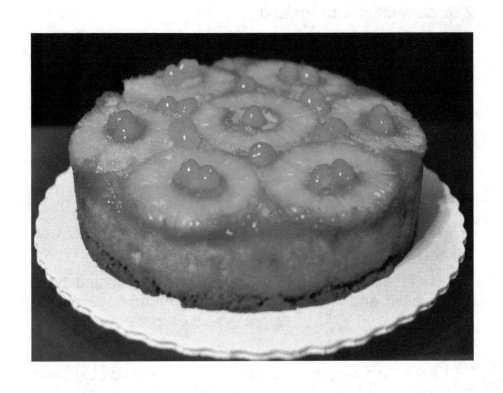

Yummy Moon Pie

Cook Time:

30 minutes

Servings:4

Ingredients:

4 graham cracker sheets, snapped in half

8 large marshmallows

8 squares each of dark, milk, and white chocolate

Directions:

1.Arrange the crackers on a cutting board. Put 2 marshmallows onto half of the graham cracker halves.

2.Place 2 squares of chocolate on top of the crackers with marshmallows.

3.Put the remaining crackers on top to create 4 sandwiches. Wrap each one in baking paper, so it resembles a parcel.

4.Bake in the preheated air fryer for 5 minutes at 340 F. Serve at room temperature or chilled. Enjoy!

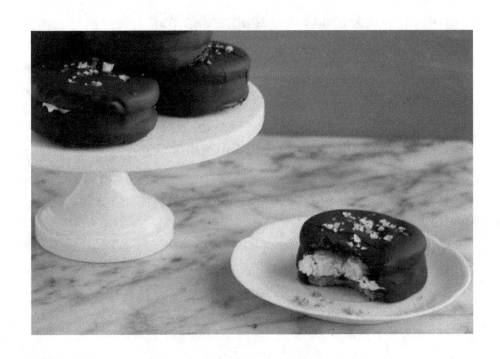

No Flour Lime Cupcakes

Cook Time:

30 minutes

Servings:4

Ingredients:

2 eggs + 1 egg yolk

Juice and zest of

1 lime

1 cup yogurt

¼ cup superfine sugar

8 oz cream cheese

1 tsp vanilla extract

Directions:

1.Preheat air fryer to 300 F. In a bowl, mix yogurt and cream cheese until uniform.

2.In another bowl, beat eggs, egg yolk, sugar, vanilla, lime juice, and zest.

3.Gently fold the in the cheese mixture. Divide the batter between greased muffin tins. Bake in the fryer for 15 minutes until golden. Serve chilled.

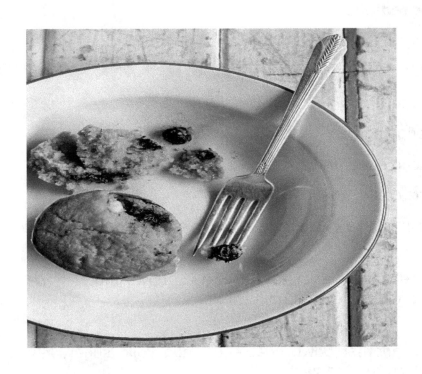

Fruit Skewers

Cook Time:

30 minutes

Servings: 2

Ingredients:

1 cup blueberries

1 banana, sliced

1 mango, peeled and cut into cubes

1 peach, cut into wedges

2 kiwi fruit, peeled and quartered

2 tbsp caramel sauce

DIRECTIONS:

1.Preheat air fryer to 340 F. Thread the fruit through your skewers.

2.Transfer to the greased frying basket and Air Fry for 6-8 minutes, turning once until the fruit caramelize slightly. Drizzle with the caramel sauce and serve. Enjoy!

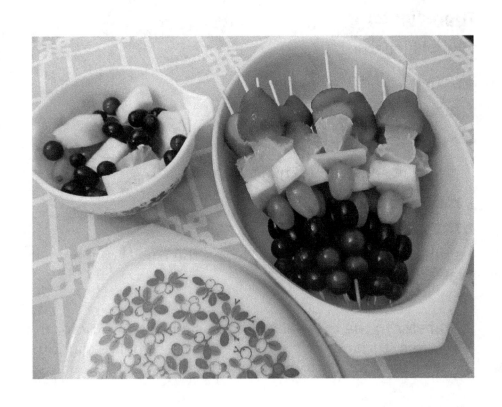

CPSIA information can be obtained
at www.ICGtesting.com
Printed in the USA
BVHW052234090521
606929BV00004B/112